To Michael & Pam
For you, your family &
client –
Dave Safely

Senior Driving Dilemmas

LIFESAVING STRATEGIES

By David Bernstein, MD   *Feb 2023*

www.davidbernsteinmd.com

Author of:

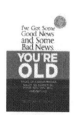

D1563648

I've Got Some Good News and Some Bad News YOU'RE OLD
Tales of a Geriatrician; What to Expect in your 60's, 70's 80's and Beyond
And
Notes on Living Longer

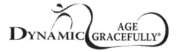

Senior Driving Dilemmas   LIFESAVING STRATEGIES
Copyright © by David Bernstein, MD

Published in the United States by Dynamic Learning

ISBN-13: 978-0-9907087-4-2
ISBN-13: 978-0-9907087-3-5 electronic version

Books are available in quantity for promotional or premium branded corporate use.
For more information on discounts, terms and media requests contact:

Dynamic Learning
Media Department
314 Shore Dr. E. Oldsmar, Florida 34677-3916
Melissa@davidbernsteinmd.com

Visit us at www.davidbernsteinmd.com

Author's Note

In order to protect the privacy of those mentioned in this book, names and certain identifying characteristics of all of the individuals whose medical histories have been described have been changed.

Furthermore, all stories are written following HIPPA (Health Portability Act of 1966) compliance guidelines.

Acknowledgements

I am grateful for the efforts of my collaborative term who worked hard to help with the publication of this book: Kathleen Smith for editing, Joyce Frustaci and Annie Mayberry for graphic designs. My wife and publicist Melissa, who has work tirelessly to help make this book a success.

In addition, I am grateful to my patients who have provided the motivation to write and who have provided the enlightenment about the trials and tribulation of aging.

I owe particular gratitude to my supporters that provided recommendation to this manuscript: Mary Dee Snow, Richard Maza, M.D., Vince Piccolo and Joanne Scott, R.N.

GET MY FREE EBOOK-
"NOTES ON LIVING LONGER"
www.davidbernsteinmd.com

Table of Contents

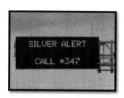

Elder Driving: When it's Time to Stop

I would like to share a little bit about myself, and my views on life, as I approach the very serious topic of driving. As a baby boomer growing up in the sixties and seventies, I was highly influenced by television and the cinema. I envisioned myself becoming a doctor and thus was a fan of several on TV – most notably the young and handsome Dr. Kildare and the gentle and kind Dr. Marcus Welby. I was equally enamored with detectives such as Lt. Colombo for his way of solving crimes and Inspector Clouseau for his clumsy, but lucky efforts in investigating law-breaking. I realized that all of the "famous" detectives in popular media were solving crimes, not only for the benefit of the victim but also for the greater good of their society. For example, when Lt. Colombo made a nuisance of himself by asking the same question over and over and then saying "now just one more question." He was often trying to bring closure to a family grief-stricken by the loss of a loved one or the theft of a cherished keepsake. Society at large benefitted from the TV detectives' successes in that it prevented the perpetrator from repeating his or her crime. Later, I felt a certain affinity for character Monk, and his tenacity for solving a crime, even when his Obsessive Compulsive Disorder (OCD) got in the way. I do not believe that I have OCD, but I do find that I can be just as tenacious in trying to solve a similarly difficult medical dilemma.

As I see it, my job as a physician is similar to that of a detective. I am in a position to use my deductive skills (some of which I learned by watching my favorite TV detectives) to solve a medical or psychological problem. My effort is for the good of my patient (and their family members), but I also look at my patients as a small but important society, whose quality of life I want to improve.

As a speaker and writer, I work to communicate with individuals and encourage them to bring about change in their lives. At the same time, I work toward making our society healthier and safer.

I have written this book because I want to help people. I want to enable them to understand that the subject of senior driving is complex and that unraveling the nuances of the problem may require the skills of a detective and the patience and understanding of a physician. The dilemma of seniors driving requires the utmost compassion and understanding, especially on the driver's family members, who must tread carefully, to provide "tough love" for the safety of their senior driver and the other drivers or pedestrians on the roadways. In this book, I will site many examples from news items and my own professional experiences.

The Alert....

I have been driving to work on the same road for several years. One day I noticed a large new sign being erected. It is the kind I am accustomed to seeing on the interstate giving advice about driving conditions, delays, and Amber Alerts. On my way to the hospital one morning, I looked up at the sign and read, "Silver Alert: Maroon Buick Century 2002 License plate PST-245". My brain snapped to attention wondering if it might be one of my patients who had become lost while driving.

As I stepped on the accelerator on my way to make rounds, I instinctively knew what had happened to prompt this Silver Alert. I pondered if the outcome would be similar to a story I had read about a few years earlier in which an elderly woman had disappeared in a town just south of Clearwater, Florida. After she had disappeared, her car was not found, nor was there any police or hospital report of an accident or injury. She was either lost hundreds of miles away from home or had driven off the road and died. A few days later, my fear was confirmed as I read the following headline in the St. Petersburg Times: "Woman, car, found in water".

The article reported that the woman had moved to be closer to her family and had been living in an adult retirement facility. The family described her as being very self-sufficient, but she had had short-term memory problems. For the first month after she moved to the new community, they had taken away her car keys "until she settled in." After 30 days, her keys were given back to her. A family member interviewed in the article indicated that "did not usually drive far from home, she just ran a few errands. We never questioned her driving skills.

We never had to have a conversation about how to take the car away because it never came up." This is a situation that we have heard over and over again. As you read further, it is my goal that I provide a clearer view of the issues that surround Senior Driving Dilemmas, while gaining insight to the problems and lifesaving strategies that may be applied as guidance in any situation related to Senior drivers.

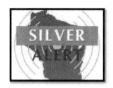

Chapter 1 – The Problem

In July 2003, an 86-year-old man drove his 1982 Buick into a crowd of pedestrians shopping at an open-air farmers market in Santa Monica, California, killing 10 and injuring more than 50 people.

In October 2005, a 93-year-old man struck a pedestrian in St. Petersburg, Florida, and did not notice the body hanging out his windshield until a tollbooth operator stopped him.

Shocking incidents such as these have reinvigorated a long-simmering debate over the risks of older drivers on the road and has led to calls for stricter state licensing policies for these drivers. The issue is particularly important in light of this demographic projection:

By 2025, drivers 65 and older will represent 25 percent of the driving population (as compared to 15 percent in 2001). (1)

Scientific studies show that physical and cognitive degeneration at older ages compromises driving ability; it is not clear just how much more dangerous older drivers are than other drivers. Most published research shows that accidents per mile driven increase when drivers are in their fifties. And, by the time people reach their eighties, accidents per mile driven are almost as high as they are for the youngest drivers. (2)

As a geriatrician, I have personally encountered situations reflective of this data. Joe was one of those situations. A retired government lawyer from the Washington, D.C. area, he and his wife lived comfortably on a government pension. They enjoyed ballroom dancing and participated in competitions frequently, spending a lot of money on the clothes required for these competitions.

Joe suffered from Addison's disease. It also appeared that he had some connective tissue condition indicated by ears that were pinned close to the skull and very hard to the touch. After I had been treating him for many years, he developed Alzheimer's disease. As is typically the case, he kept his memory and cognitive decline a secret from his wife. Eventually however, it became apparent to her as well.

What I have observed and been told by my patients, is that when friends begin to notice signs and symptoms of dementia, a diagnosis is confirmed, "they drop you like a hot potato." Fearing that this would happen, the couple kept their secret to themselves, not even discussing it with their daughter.

When the symptoms of Dementia became clear to me, we had a thorough discussion about the disease process, as well as a new medication, Cognex that had just become available. During a subsequent office visit, I strongly advised Joe and his wife that driving at this point would be dangerous and that he should relinquish his license. Each time I brought this to their attention, he refused the advice, and his wife continued to be supportive of him and his continued driving. Since I was so unsure about how to handle this issue at the time, I recalled another patient, William, from a few years earlier. His disease had progressed, and he had become even more belligerent on the topic. In light of this, I was reluctant to pursue the issue more vigorously.

Some weeks after an office visit, I received a call from Joe's wife saying that her husband had been in a serious auto accident and taken to the county trauma center. He had suffered a broken pelvis, a punctured lung, and a severe head injury. There were no injuries in the accident. Joe died five days later. While I was relieved that no one else was hurt, his wife was distraught with grief about her loss and was forever guilt-ridden that she had not followed my recommendation that her husband relinquish his license. By reflecting on these two situations, it was apparent that it is my responsibility to be more proactive with patients and families to prevent this unfortunate and preventable outcome.

I've noticed over the years that families aren't always aware that their elderly loved ones have become dangerous on the road. This circumstance may be due to a lack of information, geographical or emotional distances between family members. Some elderly drivers may remain in denial over the deterioration of the driving skills, and may hide it. The desire to remain independent is a strong one with many seniors, and the ability to drive freely is inextricably bound up with that. Also, there is just a general ignorance among Americans of all ages about the dangers of elder driving. But the risk is real, and it can result, not just in loss of life or injury, but in financial catastrophe as well.

Recently, I came across one such tragic incident while speaking to a colleague of mine in Miami, Florida. She was working with a woman who needed help supervising her elderly parents. They had retired from jobs in the private sector and were supporting themselves on social security benefits and modest pensions. This couple owned their condo and had at least $500,000 of assets invested in mutual funds. The father had several health problems that required medical attention, as did the mother, but she had psychiatric problems as well that required mood-altering medications. Neither parent had significant impairments in their driving abilities. One morning, the mother was driving on a very busy road in town and failed to yield while making a left turn. She drove directly into the path of an oncoming motorcyclist. A collision occurred, the mother was not injured, but the motorcyclist was gravely injured, and died soon after arrival at the hospital.

The mother was distraught, but she eventually recovered from the stress of the accident and her insurance company paid the claim to the motorcyclist's family. The deceased's family also filed a civil wrongful death lawsuit against the parents of the client, thus threatening the assets the retired couple had acquired over the course of their working careers. The father and mother who had sacrificed all of their lives for retirement are soon to declare bankruptcy. They will likely lose all their savings and will have to survive on social security. An additional tragedy is the loss of whatever inheritance the daughter would have assumed had the accident not happened.

While this individual *may* have been impaired by her illness or her medication, this incident serves as an example of the financial and social ramifications of <u>any</u> adult's responsibilities related to an accident, and the subsequent disability or loss of life. When we know someone should not be driving and don't take action, the guilt and responsibility spreads to include us all. Let's look at some sobering facts that may help us in the future accept the challenge and provide guidance to influence a senior from continuing driving.

How big is the problem? What are the Facts?

"In 2012, more than 5,560 older adults were killed and more than 214,000 injured in motor vehicle crashes. These statistics reveal that an average of 15 older adults killed and 556 injured in crashes every day". (3)

Today there are more seniors on the roads than ever. In 2012 there were an estimated 36 million licensed older drivers on the road, which represents a 34 percent increase since 1999. (4)

Per mile traveled; fatal crash rates increase starting at age 75, and increase notably after age 80. This fatality rate is largely due to increased susceptibility to injury and medical complications among older drivers, rather than an increased tendency to get into crashes.

The age-related decline in vision and cognitive functioning (the ability to reason and remember), as well as physical changes, may affect some older adults' driving abilities. Across all age groups, males had substantially higher death rates than females.

There are some existing protective factors that already improve older drivers' safety.
They include:
High incidence of seat belt use- More than three in every four (77%) of surviving older motor vehicle occupants (drivers and passengers) involved in crashes with fatalities were wearing seat belts at the time of the crash, compared to 63% for other adult occupants (18 to 64 years of age). The tendency to drive when conditions are the safest- Older drivers tend to limit their driving during bad weather and at night and drive fewer miles than younger drivers.

Lower incidence of impaired driving- older adult drivers are less likely to drink and drive than other adult drivers. Only 5% of older drivers involved in fatal crashes had a blood alcohol concentration (BAC) of 0.08 grams per deciliter (g/dl) or higher, compared to 25% of drivers between the ages of 21 and 64 years. (4)

Older adults can take further steps to stay safe on the road, including:

1. Exercise regularly to increase strength and flexibility
2. Ask your doctor or pharmacist to review medicines, both prescription and over-the-counter, to reduce side effects and interactions.
3. Have your eyes checked by an eye doctor at least once a year. Wear glasses and corrective lenses as required.
4. Drive only during daylight hours and in good weather.
5. Find the safest route with well-lit streets, intersections with left turn arrows, and easy parking.
6. Plan your route before you drive.
7. Leave a large following distance behind the car in front of you.
8. Avoid distractions in your car such as listening to a loud radio, talking on your cell phone, texting, and eating.
9. Consider using potential alternatives to driving to get around, such as riding with a friend or using public transit.

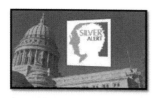

Chapter 2 – What to do now?

Several years ago, when I began observing the problem with senior driving, I contacted one of my patients who had had a long career at the Department of Motor Vehicles (DMV). She informed me that the DMV has a form that anyone could fill out to anonymously report an unsafe driver. When the DMV receives such a report, they notify the individual and require him or her to submit a form to their doctor. The process places the onus on the physician to verify whether or not the individual should be driving. The doctor's opinion and involvement are important in this process. At the time, I didn't feel that I had the technical skills to determine whether or not someone should drive. My knowledge and clinical reasoning led me to believe that a patient with diminished physical and/or cognitive abilities cannot be safe behind the wheel of a car. This danger would be the case for themselves and all other drivers on the road. I have used this form many times anonymously reporting unsafe drivers. As a result many unsafe drivers have had their licenses revoked.

According to the Florida Department of Highway Safety and Motor Vehicles, research indicates that most people will outlive their driving ability by about ten years. The most at-risk driver is the one with cognitive impairment. The American Medical Association (AMA) regards the safety of older drivers as a public health issue. They estimate that the per-mile fatality rate for drivers over 85-years old is nine times as great as drivers 25 to 69 years old.

Why is relinquishing a driver's license such a problem? Why are our elderly taking such risks, not only for themselves but also for their loved ones and others on the road? What do they see when they look in the mirror? I have been pondering these questions for many years and continue to be amazed at the resistance I receive when broaching the subject of the "senior driving dilemma."

In my years as a geriatrician, the reactions, and subsequent behaviors I observe after a discussion on the topic of driving are not so surprising. Consider this: these seniors are fighting to maintain their independence. For some, the last bastion of that independence is their ability to drive. When they can no longer get back and forth to the doctor, grocery store or hairdresser, they may view life as being over. They might have to move to a retirement center to access transportation or, even worse, move to a different town or state to be near one of their children, an option that most find totally unacceptable. Many of them might willingly take advice from one of their children about some things, but giving up their driving is not one of them.

Another factor to consider is a lack of historical precedence. The group of elders who are currently facing the issue of when to quit driving lived through the Great Depression and WWII. Many people had cars during and after the depression but in not nearly the numbers that acquired them after WWII (during the mid-1940s through the 1950s). As a group, this cohort did not have to confront their parents about relinquishing driving privileges. For the most part, their parents did not have the life expectancy that we enjoy today, so the kinds of conversations we are discussing here simply did not take place.

When I talk to my older patients about how they have dealt with their parents on this issue, they frequently tell me that their mothers did not drive, so they faced only one-half of the problem. Most of the time, their fathers were still driving when they got sick or suffered a stroke and then just stopped. This demographic is the first generation of individuals who face this issue. Senior driving and the decisions that surround their continued safety is uncharted territory.

In a survey conducted among baby boomers for the website caring.com in partnership with The National Safety Council, investigators found that suggesting to parents that they stop driving was considered to be the most difficult subject for children to bring up with their parents. They found this to be a subject more difficult even than discussing funeral wishes or selling the family home! Thirty-nine percent (39%) of those surveyed said they would not be comfortable discussing driving status with their parents, while 25% felt that their parents should voluntarily impose some restrictions or safeguards on themselves.

It's a fact that public transportation systems in most cities in this country do not meet most travelers' needs, and that goes for seniors also. They are "spoiled" in this respect; when they want to go somewhere, they just get in the car and go. The prospect of calling a cab and waiting to be picked up is just unacceptable. Many do rely on friends for rides but express that they do not like to impose and, as a result, they often become either isolated or very dependent on others.

Solving this problem is difficult and requires a solid understanding of the personalities and needs of each. Love and respect from children and friends are imperative, as is providing alternatives when terminating driving and taking the car keys. We have dangerous drivers on our roadways that are in total denial that they have lost the skill to drive safely, and they are unable to determine when to stop. As a society and as family members, we have been too timid in addressing this critical problem. As a result, lives are put in jeopardy every day.

Are New Policies Needed?

Medical research has demonstrated that as people age their driving ability becomes impaired. The most common problem is declining eyesight. Glaucoma, macular degeneration, and cataracts, all of which become more common with age, reduce night and peripheral vision and vision acuity, and cause individuals to become more sensitive to glare. Impaired vision is strongly associated with a greater likelihood of causing an accident among older drivers.

Studies have shown that normal changes in brain function due to aging may slow reflex reactions and reduce the ability to take in information from disparate sources simultaneously. More severe changes in brain functioning, such as depression and dementia, as well as the use of medications to treat those illnesses, may seriously hamper an older person's ability to drive. Other common afflictions among older people such as heart disease, arthritis, and insomnia, can also affect driving skills.

There is also evidence that some older individuals compensate for their impairment by changing their driving behavior. Many older drivers drive less frequently, and, when they do drive, they tend to avoid high-speed zones and driving at night. Eventually, most older adults decide to stop driving altogether, either because they recognize that they are likelier to cause an accident, or because a family member or doctor urges them to stop driving. In determining the appropriate policy for older drivers, self-regulation must be taken into account.

The lessons here are serious. Over the next 20 years, there will be an astounding growth in senior drivers in the United States. The population of adults over 75 years old will grow from 18 million to 31 million. Since the accident rate for drivers over the age of 65 is higher than for any group other than teenagers, this could account for 100,000 accidents in the next 20 years.

New approaches are being developed as information accumulates about the growing risk this population faces. The American Medical Association, in conjunction with the National Highway Traffic Safety Administration, has created a guide booklet for physicians who treat older drivers.

The Physician's Guide to Assessing and Counseling Older Drivers is available online at www.ama-assn.org or geriatricscareonline.org/ProductAbstract/physicians-guide-to-assessing-and-counseling-older-drivers/B013.

As an aid to empower caregivers and families, The Hartford Financial Services group and the Massachusetts Institute of Technology has developed a 30-page booklet called *At the Crossroads*. The booklet facilitates conversation about driving cessation, independently, or in classrooms.

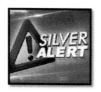

Chapter 3 – Taking the Keys

As a physician, I take my responsibility for the management of my patients' care very seriously in all areas. When addressing safety I do not limit my evaluation just to driving, nor should children or aging parents. Reducing falls, especially when they are the result of hazardous activity, is high up on my list of concerns. Having a patient's home evaluated for trip hazards, such as throw rugs and electrical cords, is essential. And I advise all my patients to cease going up ladders and to stop using step stools – a fall from either one can result in serious, if not life-threatening, injuries.

I also have a personal view of the universe. It suggests that if I see something in my community, I know that the same drama is probably unfolding in every city and community in this country, and the world, for that matter. So, if I am aware of an unsafe driver in my town, there are likely also others in cities x, y and z.

Over my career as a physician, I have faced the issue of impaired drivers countless times. It is always a painful experience. The discussion triggers tears, anger and, sometimes, people demonstrating an outright disregard for the law, or for others who share the roadways. When my children were young, and I knew that these horribly unsafe drivers were on the local roads I felt very uneasy. I still do.

As with many experiences I have had in my career, there is both good news and bad news. While I was writing my first book, *I've Got Some Good News and Some Bad News; YOU'RE OLD*, I asked a friend for some feedback on my chapter about driving. I approached this friend because, even though Samuel was a successful building contractor, he had majored in journalism at college. I was also well aware that his aging mother had Alzheimer's disease and should not be driving. I handed Samuel my polished chapter and then my wife and I gave him a short lecture on the subject. We waited just a few weeks for his response.

When I next saw Samuel and his wife at a social event several weeks later, he told me about the impact the chapter had had on him. Samuel and his brother had discussed the chapter and then firmly told their mother that she would no longer be driving. The conversation was not an easy one, and his very proud mother put up quite a fuss. But, in the end, it all worked out. Today, the mother is still alive and well and no longer driving. My wife and I get an amazing feeling of satisfaction when we think that we might have saved a life or two by speaking to Samuel about his mother's driving.

In my book, I also refer to a patient named Russ, who struggled to make a decision about moving to a retirement community after his wife, Marge, became seriously ill.

While Marge was in rehab, she was adamant that she did not want to move into an assisted living facility as it would have meant living away from her husband, Russ. The couple resolved to stay together and vehemently resisted attempts by staff at her rehab facility and her doctor to separate them. Ultimately, they made a decision and compromised, getting a full-time aide to move into their modest two-bedroom apartment in an independent living facility. Despite my predictions of doom and gloom, they have thrived well beyond my wildest expectations. This example has reminded me to be more open-minded and creative in arriving at the safest, most appropriate option for my patients who are in decline.

Much to my chagrin, even with a full-time live-in aide who was capable of driving his nearly brand new red Cadillac, Russ insisted on continuing to drive. He had nowhere he had to go.

He just wanted to make trips to the pharmacy and grocery store. But, as far as I was concerned, Russ was unnecessarily risking his life. I was familiar with the area in which he lived and knew how treacherous it could be to handle the left turns needed to negotiate even a short trip to the local drug store. Russ has moderate symptoms of Parkinson's disease, meaning his gait is slow and unsteady, and his balance is poor, all of which put him at high risk for a fall. Also, his reflexes have slowed considerably. It seemed inconceivable to me that Russ would even consider continuing to drive his bright red Cadillac. Nonetheless, I handed him a copy of my book and at our very next visit he informed me that after reading it, he immediately stopped driving. What a pleasant surprise for me! Providing resources, statistics and information on senior driving may not always work at the time, but it is especially helpful when encouraging someone to stop driving.

What seniors face when their driving skills progressively deteriorate underlines bigger problems. There is a failure to recognize the loss of motor skill, reflexes, and visual perception, as well as any authority that might terminate their driving privileges.

This age group has never had to deal with terminating their own parents' driving privileges. Most of their parents did not live to an advanced age nor did they suffer the chronic diseases that today's senior's face. In other words, their parents died before their driving skills deteriorated. As a result, today's elderly have never been faced with this particular problem.

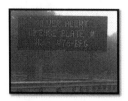

Chapter 4 - Empowerment

What I learned from Russ in the previous chapter empowered me to broach the subject with two other couples in my practice, who I was certain should no longer be driving. I planned to offer each an opportunity to take a driving examination to determine their physical and cognitive capabilities to drive.

The DriveABLE In-Office cognitive assessment (5) is an examination performed at a local health center and has been compared favorably with The DriveABLE On-Road Evaluation (DORE) in a retrospective study.(6)

The In-Office cognitive assessment consists of 6 tests: motor speed and control, span of attentional field, spatial judgment and decision making, speed of attentional shifting, executive functions, and identification of hazardous driving situations.

This In-Office cognitive assessment is completed and scored on a computer. A certified assessor provides standardized instructions and gives one to three practice trials before each test to ensure that the patient understands what it is he or she needs to do. The assessor remains with the patient throughout the evaluation. The patient responds by simply touching a touch-sensitive screen or pressing a button. Scoring and report generation are automated and a report is automatically generated based on the findings. The results are compared against norms with the outcome measure being the predicted probability of failing the DORE. I have used this test several times in the past ten years and have found it to be a very reliable test to determine the probability that an individual will pass or fail a road test.

I realized that both couples would probably feel certain they would pass the test with ease so I proposed that the results be binding and that, if they failed, they would no longer drive their cars. I was certain none of the four patients would pass and that all would have to stop driving. I was well aware of the social implications and possible reactions for each – anger, hostility, and loss of independence among them.

Two couples, two scenarios and two outcomes.

Sally and Richard have been my patients for a long time. They are former missionaries and belong to a tight community of long-time friends, many of whom are also my patients. Over the years, the pair would come in together for their medical visits. Richard kept track of their medications with a neatly typed list, fixed with scotch tape in his little black appointment book.

A few years earlier, it appeared that both Sally and Richard were slipping a bit. Their first stumble in my presence occurred when they couldn't remember where they had eaten dinner the night before. This event alerted me to start asking them a few non-threatening questions each time they came into the office; it was my informal test of their short-term memory. Within a few visits, it became clear that there was a significant problem.

For example, at one afternoon visit, the two of them couldn't recall where or what they'd had for lunch. I then determined that the medication list that Richard had been keeping in his little book included medications I had discontinued a year prior. When he complained of gastrointestinal side effects, I could not establish what medications he was taking. As a result, I could not properly evaluate his treatment. Clearly, as his physician, I was facing a complex and serious problem.

The matter got worse when Sally and Richard's friends chimed in, indicating that they too had observed the same types of memory problems in the couple. They shared their concerns about Richard's driving. Adding to the problem was the fact that the couple's son lived out of town.

When the son and I finally spoke, I discovered that he was in complete denial. He confessed that he did not think there was a problem and, if there was one, he was not the right person to intervene. Richard did all the driving; Sally had not driven a car for many years since Richard was the better driver, and her eyes were not as good as they had been. Sally served as Richard's navigator. When my suspicions increased, I started to get frustrated with this couple. I would inquire about what vehicle they drove, and they could not identify it.

When I suggested that Richard stop driving he became very angry saying that I was out of line for making the suggestion. He then left the office abruptly. The final chapter is unfinished. Sally and Richard continue to deny that they have a problem; Richard continues to drive, and both refuse to move to a more secure environment.

The second couple, Herman and Alice, were both physically frail. It has been a wonder to me that they could even get in and out of a car, no less shop for groceries or prepare a meal. They had been patients for many years, and I have treated them for almost every medical condition that I know. The list includes diabetes, hypertension, coronary artery disease, atrial fibrillation, stroke, Alzheimer's disease and Parkinson's disease. These are just the ones I have to address each time they come in for office visits. Alice had never been the driver in the family; Herman had assumed those responsibilities long ago. Alice had not driven in ten years. During that period, she had suffered a stroke, which compromised her vision when she gazed to the left side. For several years there was friction between them about issues that would challenge any happily married couple. When they discussed moving from their condo to an alternative living facility it provoked so much malice and ill will that the subject ended without resolution. In addition to the social ramifications of such a move, there were financial ones to consider as well.

Normally, when patients come to my office for a visit, my staff escorts them to the scale to measure their weight and then has them sit in a chair in the exam room. I usually greet the patient while they are sitting and carry out my visit until I have them walk to the exam table. During some visits, I have my patients walk longer distances but usually later in the visit. On this particular visit, I stood in the hallway and watched Herman and then Alice walk to the scale. I was astonished at how poorly each walked, especially Herman. Before I even entered the exam room, I gathered my thoughts. Herman, the driver, had been weaker than usual for a few weeks and, as I started to review his medications, I grew more anxious as I realized his Parkinson's had advanced. This condition was resulting in worsening balance and gait, not to mention a slowing of his reflexes. I wondered how, if there were an emergency, he would be able to move fast enough to escape a catastrophic outcome. Then I wondered about the same thing about his Alzheimer's disease, and his anemia, the multiple medications for his heart disease, and his blood pressure. "Wow," I thought, "Herman continuing to drive was a serious problem". When I shared my concerns with him, he acted as though I was addressing someone else. Alice chimed in, "But Doctor, Herman is a good driver and has never been in an accident." She added that if ever there was an issue with his driving, she could easily take over (even though she had not touched a steering wheel in ten years). Another "Wow" shot through my head. What was I to do? I was so unprepared for this type of response that I was speechless. I needed more time to collect my thoughts. I was lucky as they had a lunch appointment and had to leave before I had time to bring up the subject of their driving. Alice had booked an appointment for another week, and I would have an opportunity to address my concerns then.

During subsequent office visits with both Richard and Sally, and later with Herman and Alice, I expressed my concerns again more clearly and more emphatically. I provided each of them with an opportunity to take the DRIVEable exam to determine their competency to drive. Each agreed to abide by the results of the test. Since Sally was not interested in driving, she did not participate in the testing.

When the time came for Richard's testing, he and Sally were so confused that they missed both the appointment for the test and their visits with me the following week. Richard then told me that he had never agreed to such a bargain, and I had to bring my staff in to refute his claim. Additionally, I called the testing center where I had scheduled the test, and I discovered that Richard had never arrived to take the test. Richard subsequently backed down and agreed that perhaps he might have missed it. After that appointment, I completed paperwork to be sent to the Department of Motor Vehicles (DMV) recommending that they revoke Richard's driving privileges. Two weeks later a letter from the DMV must have arrived in Richard's mail revoking his license. He arrived at my office without an appointment asking if I had anything to do with the revocation of his license. We sat and chatted about it for some time. It was clear to me that soon Richard would completely forget about our conversation. He has continued to drive, now with a revoked license. When it eventually became clear that Sally had sometimes started driving in place of Richard, I sent paperwork to the DMV suggesting revocation of her license as well.

When Herman and Alice returned for their test results, they sat waiting for vindication and permission for Herman to continue driving. They were shocked when I revealed that Herman had scored a 99% probability of failing his road test; Alice's score was a 93% probability of failure. They had both dismally failed, yet they protested that it was an unfair test as it had utilized computer technology. The couple would have preferred having the tester on the road with them (which would have only risked the examiner's life along with theirs).

Also, they protested that their loss of independence would result in challenges to remaining in their condo. The couple's argument couldn't overcome my concern about having them risk their lives continuing to drive while also jeopardizing the lives of others. I was frustrated with them, as they had failed to plan for this eventuality or adapt by making desperately needed changes. As I met with the couple, I made my recommendation clear that I would be notifying the DMV of their test results and recommend revocation of their drivers' licenses.

There was drama. Herman was stoic, but Alice was inconsolable and in complete disbelief. I remember her telling me that she would not move, she would not hire a driver, or take a cab, or ask a friend for a ride. After they had left my office, I received several telephone calls from their children, not all supportive of my recommendation or referral to the DMV.

Over the years of my career as a physician, I have had to face this kind of situation countless times, and it is always a painful experience. The reality of losing the privilege of driving triggers tears, anger, and, sometimes, outright disregard for the law or for others who share the roadways.

Another option to consider is the AARP Smart Driver Program. (7) It is a low cost 6 hour (in Florida) program geared towards, but not limited to, senior citizens. The goal of the Smart Driver program is to keep seniors driving longer with a theme that "*Things Change- our bodies are changing, our cars are changing, our roads are changing*" explained Vince, an instructor of the course. Recognizing those changes and adapting them is what they are trying to instill in the classroom. He continued, "*We remind them that they no longer have quick reflexes, the peripheral vision, the sharp hearing, or the physical flexibility they once had, so we need to be smart in our choices as to when, where, and how we drive*".

From his experience conducting twenty classroom sessions during the previous year, Vince tells me, "*that he conducts his sessions with approximately 500 seniors, from those in their early fifties to their mid-nineties who are still driving and still sharp (but not all, unfortunately). Most take the course for the small discount on insurance they may receive. He adds that the discount lasts for three years, the tips you'll learn in this course will last you a lifetime. We're not teaching them how to drive; we're teaching them how to drive smarter*". Vince informs me, "The instruction begins with the changes in our bodies, and the effects of medical conditions, medications, and changes, some subtle, some not, in our vision, hearing, and cognitive abilities. The course stresses that the attendees become aware of and recognize these changes, and adapt driving to them. There is encouragement for a close partnership and communication with their physician and their pharmacist. The drivers learn to be aware of the effects of those medications and conditions that may have an impact on their ability to drive safely". Polling the classes, Vince has found that very few have asked their doctors about the potential impact of their prescribed medicines on their driving ability, and even fewer have had their doctor volunteer such information. This gap would suggest the potential for improvement on both sides.

The point is made in the AARP class; the person best able to evaluate driving skills is the person who sits in the seat alongside. The course recognizes that the decision to limit, or stop driving entirely, is an uncomfortable one. Vince tells me that he can sense a tension in the room- the verbal interaction which was sprightly and involved in the earlier sessions, decreases as he discusses this potentially uncomfortable topic, but it is a necessary one. *"We discuss independent driving evaluations to determine our current level of driving skill, and the importance of the evaluation to determine where changes or improvements may be made. Further, we discuss alternatives to driving if and when that should become necessary."*

Regarding the DriveAble program I mentioned earlier in this book, it is primarily geared to those who have been diagnosed with Dementia or Alzheimer's, but are in the early stages. DriveAble does not provide evaluations for the senior citizens who want an independent opinion.

Locally in Clearwater, Fl., the Suncoast Safety Council conducts driving evaluations involving both cognitive and practical review. There is a fee to take the hour and a half to two hour assessment. To me, any cost for this type of evaluation is reasonable considering the potential savings in bodily or property damage occurring from an accident. I am certain there are other sources throughout this country for independent evaluations wherever readers of this book may live.

If you have a loved one whose driving skills are putting him or her and others on the road at risk, please do not put off the conversation that you know you must have with them. It is my recommendation that you also include the family physician in these conversations. We want to help.

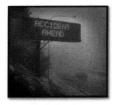

Chapter 5 – Solutions

There are several expressions that I love. They come to my mind often many times during a work week as I focus on making the lives of my patients better. One is a quote from the fictional character, Hannibal Smith, who was the leader of the "A" Team on the television show of the same name. He would say, "I love it when a plan comes together." I use the expression after a plan with many complex moving parts falls into place resulting in the desired outcome. I appreciate having the challenge of dealing with complex problems. These types of problems allow me to use the observational and reasoning skills I have developed over the years. These patient situations afford me the opportunity to see the faces of grateful patients when favorable outcomes occur.

Additionally, I love hearing my favorite five-word expression, "Doctor Bernstein, you were right." Those five words are sweet to hear from patients who challenge my judgment and years of experience every step of the way. I know I am not a psychic, but there are times when it appears that way. What happens is a combination of the wisdom I have gained in my practice of more than 30 years and my reference points of previous experiences. This combination is much like the forecasting ability of my local meteorologist.

Samuel, the building contractor I mentioned in Chapter 3, read the chapter about driving in my book, ***I've Got Some Good News and Some Bad News; YOU'RE OLD***. (8) Upon completing the chapter and had an intervention with his mother,

Phyllis. It was a challenging confrontation for Samuel because his mother is a very bright woman, a retired social worker. She was able to refuse her adult children's request that she no longer drive. Fortunately, she also had sufficient assets to be able to move into a very nice independent living facility that was close to her family and where transportation was available. Lucky for me Phyllis was not my patient, and I served only as a knowledgeable friend giving advice to Samuel and his family.

As a physician, I applied a great deal of pressure on Herman and Alice. Both became very angry when I informed them that they had both failed the computerized testing. I made many suggestions including; getting full-time help at home, using a taxi service or a local driver for daily errands, or moving to an independent living facility.

They agonized over making a decision and were unable to commit to any. Alice made a separate visit to my office with her son to discuss the unfairness of the situation. She shed many tears because of the predicament "her doctor" created. When I tried to save her further embarrassment by withholding notification to the DMV, she challenged me, demanding that I send in the final paperwork for revocation of her license. Her intention was to demand a hearing with the DMV to retain her license. I obliged and sent in the paperwork.

Within a few weeks, my staff noticed that when either Herman or Alice came to my office for their medical visits, they were accompanied by another man in his 60s; presumably he was a driver. I am certain the couple harbor resentment towards me about their predicament, but they remain alive and safe in the condo they enjoy so much. At least they still feel a degree of independence.

The challenges associated with Richard and Sally had me using all of my skills. I was required to be a doctor, a social worker, and an enforcer, all at the same time. I made calls to the couple's son in New York, and discussed the situation with concerned friends, all the while respecting everyone's privacy and health insurance privacy accountability rules. My office was open to both, and they took advantage of the fact by dropping in unannounced to ask about medication, or what I meant when I told them that Richard should not be driving. Because of the frequent visits to my office, my entire office staff, working as a team, was aware of their situation, and we maintained consistency in dealing with them. After the revocation of Richard's license, he continued to drive. When I told him that he must stop, he had Sally drive. I then reported her to the DMV and requested that they revoke her license. When the initial letter from the DMV arrived, Richard drove immediately to my office to raise a ruckus. But, by the time he registered in my office, he had already forgotten his intention. Eventually, two years after being contacted, Richard and Sally's son became more involved in the drama and encouraged Richard and Sally to get ready to move into an assisted living facility. Lucky for everyone involved there has been no traffic accidents.

Here's another good news story. I have been taking care of Jane for a long time, at least twenty years. I first met her when I admitted her to the hospital after a fall in which she suffered a spinal compression fracture. Over the years, I have treated her for high blood pressure, coronary artery disease and high cholesterol. Despite having a weakened heart and requiring a pacemaker and defibrillator, she thrived living the life of a widow. She took excellent care of herself, did all her cooking and cleaning and most of her shopping. And she had friends who would occasionally shop for her. Jane had boasted about visiting Hawaii over twenty times and loved to tell me stories about those trips, including going to see Don Ho perform and meeting him backstage. She became frail in such a gradual way that I had lost sight of how difficult it had become for her to continue all of her daily activities. I recommended that she consider moving back to Michigan to be closer to her family, but she declined. She reminded me that she still loved driving her

13-year-old PT Cruiser; it was one of the few joys she had left. When she told me that, I stifled the urge to shout, "Yikes!" Jane was certain that, at age 94, there was nothing that could hinder her driving or living independently.

Jane had always been plagued by back pain and in recent months her pain had intensified. I offered to send the best massage therapist in town (Mary Dee, who also happens to have a Ph.D. in psychology) to her home to see if massage treatments would help her back. Her back was so bad that the improvements were marginal. After three of four treatments with this therapist, Jane returned to my office and told me that she had put her condo up for sale and had already accepted an offer. And she would stop driving because she intended to move to Michigan in three weeks. I was disappointed that she would be leaving my practice after so many years but very pleased that she had decided to sell her PT Cruiser and stop driving. I asked her how she finally decided to stop driving and move, and she told me, "I'm just taking Mary Dee's advice."

Susan has been a patient only a few years as her former physician retired, and she chose me to continue providing her care. She was in her mid-eighties, had multiple medical problems and had a recent mild stroke. She was a widow for many years and valued her independence. Susan worked in real estate late into her seventies, had been frugal all her life, and made all of her decisions. She was a proud woman. After her stroke she noted she had problems controlling her urine and bowels and found herself more isolated. She had been driving for more than sixty years and after the stroke she had been advised by her Physical Therapists not to drive. The determined individual that she was she decided to test her ability and drove several times before making her first visit to me since her stroke.

At that visit, she announced to me quite proudly that she had moved to the retirement facility I had recommended to her over a year prior. She confessed that she was so happy there that she should have done in years earlier. When I asked her what precipitated the move, she explained that she felt very uncomfortable behind the wheel and had to stop driving. By living in this particular retirement community, she no longer had to drive for groceries or to go out to dinner. Is this an example of "I love it when a plan comes together", or "Dr. Bernstein, you were right"?

In the next chapter you will find some valuable scripts for dealing with some specific circumstances, which occur all too frequently in families with senior driver dilemmas.

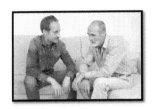

Chapter 6 – Some Scripts for Intervention

"Suspect everyone, trust no one"—Inspector Clouseau

This is one of the mantras I use when I am evaluating my older adult patients. I encourage family members and friends to gather as much information as possible before intervening. Has there been a traffic citation, an auto accident, a fender bender, or recent and suspicious bodywork on the senior's car? Have there been attempts to hide this kind of evidence from family?

If so, contact the senior's physician's office, report your concerns and try to determine if the staff shares your suspicions as well. Determine if the physician is prepared to ask for a driving evaluation or report the erratic driving to the DMV. Anyone can initiate the delicate process of getting an individual to relinquish a driver's license and no one should back off for fear of repercussions. If you are a family member and love the individual, if you are a neighbor and care about the wellbeing of a dear friend, or if you work in a facility where you have seen someone who demonstrates poor judgment or poor motor skills, you should be involved in the process. A team approach adds to the potential for success when addressing the problem of an unsafe senior driver.

Sometimes it can be difficult to get clear perspective on the issue at hand. In the section that follows I have presented four different scenarios that might provide a starting point for considering intervention options. The reader might find one or a combination of several that applies to their particular challenge.

Scenario #1

Parents are independent and financially secure

This situation can be a real challenge because they have and always will hold all the purse strings and could intimate or outright threaten a future inheritance action. In this event make it clear that you love them and it is not about the money. Let them know you want them to enjoy all the money they have worked so long and hard to save and that it could be used for transportation. Use the story about the couple who had to file for bankruptcy when the wife was responsible for the death of the motorcyclist. Let them know that they have been wonderful, upstanding citizens, and ask how they would like to go to their graves knowing that one false move late in life tarnished their years of great citizenship. Have them imagine the embarrassment to family and friends if their status and reputation changed as a result of one bad choice in life.

Scenario #2

Out of town parents and difficult transportation alternatives

The discussion about this kind of situation should take place face to face so body language can be interpreted. Often, parents are in a different city from their children, and sometimes it's specifically to avoid interference from their children. It may be part of the older adults' plan or modus operandi. Be armed with all the facts and options when you arrive to speak with them; be prepared to answer every question or objection. Be prepared to offer to move them to your city, or to a local independent living facility where transportation is provided, or provide a home health care option with a ride service or taxi service. By giving up the car they will save on the cost of gasoline and auto insurance (which is high among the elderly, especially if a claim has been made). I often hear, "I have never been in an accident or had a violation!" Don't buy it. The past does not necessarily reflect future events.

Scenario #3

Major medical condition resulting in generalized weakness and debility

Here, I would stress that they don't need to be going places in the condition they are in. They should have someone else do their shopping. What if they had a flat tire or accident; how would they handle a situation in which they would have to be in and out of the car? In their condition it could be stressful and could potentially negatively affect their health conditions resulting in hospitalization with additional rehab, or death. Suggest that they might have a milestone event to look forward to in the near future —a wedding, an anniversary or birthday.

Scenario #4

Dementia or Parkinson's disease

This is a tough problem, as it is very hard to be logical with adults who have these types of neurologic problems. You may feel frustrated for not attending to problem earlier when they may have been more reasonable. I strongly suggest you beg, borrow and steal, using all suggestions provided so far in the previous scenarios.

Consider an intervention in which all of the family confronts the unsafe driver. The intervention may end up resembling a negotiation session with terrorists, or teenagers, whichever you consider more difficult. Your logic will never be their logic. Enlist assistance from a physician, have the senior driver reported to DMV and offer to pay for the senior's transportation, or take them to local assisted living facilities to see if it could appeal to them.

Here are some thoughts that may apply to your particular situation. But, feel free to come up with your own ideas to use as a guide or support as you move forward with your plan.

Begin with the end result or goal in mind: _Senior Not Driving_. Anticipate instituting a taxi service or a move to a location where driving is not necessary or when there are family members to do all the driving.

You're dealing with an elder or parent(s) — treat them with love and respect. Treat them like the adults they are. But if they do act like children, you might have to resort to treating them as such using methods similar to those you used on your children.

Understand what is motivating them to be so stubborn. It may be possible to address the reason for the behavior or offer a trade. For example, "when you give up driving you will have an opportunity to eat dinner with our family more often and sleep over."

I have met some people who are proud of their ethnic roots, which might include being incredibly stubborn. These people would cut off their nose to spite their face and I don't really know how to deal with them. You might have to take an extreme position and force the issue.

Accept that this is a common situation; it is painful but must be addressed — you are a big boy/girl.

Being coercive is acceptable to get to the end result. This is a bit like employing Jewish guilt: motivate with promises around future events. By doing this you might have an even better chance of attending your grandchild's graduation or wedding.

Be prepared to retreat, only to try again.

Be prepared to accept the things you just cannot change, and not beat yourself up if you don't succeed.

Use teamwork; ask other family members and close friends for help. Contact the primary care doctor's office for advice; accept counsel and the support of others when you have setbacks.

It is clear that older age and driving is an extremely emotionally charged issue and one that all of us, regardless of our situation, need to take seriously. If we are young adults raising a family, the older impaired driver may pose a risk to our loved ones. As we enter middle age, our parents might become unsafe drivers and this sensitive subject will need to be broached. The sooner we feel comfortable discussing the issue and laying the groundwork for a future discussion, the better we will be prepared when for the moment when action needs to be taken. For the older adult reading this book, please consider your own safety and driving skills.

As the aging driver or the child of a parent whose skills have deteriorated, we are reluctant to broach the subject, largely due to its implication of submission to physical or cognitive decline. In addition, older adults are faced with a change in status within their community and a subsequent perception of incompetence. As a society, and as individuals, we must all, not only take responsibility for ourselves, but for our loved ones who are taking risks with their own lives and the lives of others.

Attitudes change slowly. This book is devoted to changing attitudes about senior driving, one reader at a time. It is not just my personal crusade; it belongs to all of us, for the sake of our parents and our children and grandchildren.

There are positive notes here. Done with compassion and love, driving cessation could bring about a sense of relief, not only for the children of the unsafe driver, but for the driver himself or herself. They might feel the huge burden and responsibility of driving lifted from their shoulders. It could bring family members together, getting them to share responsibilities for transportation and provide more time for generations to spend with each other.

After reading this book I urge the reader to take action where needed. Talk with your family. Speak with health care providers to get their insights. Have testing performed in just the same way you would order an EKG (Electrocardiograph), chest x-ray, MRI (Magnetic Resonance Imaging), or CT (Computer Tomography) scan. Take the test results seriously and follow the recommendations of professionals. The process might be difficult, but the outcome may save lives.

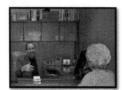

Photo taken by Melissa Bernstein

To a Long and Healthy Life...

David Bernstein, MD

References

(1) What Risks Do Older Drivers Pose to Traffic Safety?
http://www.rand.org/pubs/research_briefs/RB9272/index1.htm l)

(2) Reuben, D. B., Silliman, R. A. and Traines, M. (1988), **The Aging Driver Medicine, Policy, and Ethics.** *Journal of the American Geriatrics Society, 36: 1135-1142. doi: 10.1111/j.1532-5415.1988.tb04403.x*

(3) Injury Prevention & Control: Motor Vehicle Safety
http://www.cdc.gov/motorvehiclesafety/older_adult_drivers/

(4) Injury Prevention & Control: Motor Vehicle Safety
http://www.cdc.gov/motorvehiclesafety/older_adult_drivers/

(5) The DriveABLE Cognitive Assessment Tool
http://driveable.com/index.php/products/in-office

(6) Accuracy of the DriveABLE cognitive assessment to determine cognitive fitness to drive . Allen R. Dobbs, PhD
http://www.cfp.ca/content/59/3/e156.full

(7) AARP Smart Drive Program,
http://www.aarpdriversafety.org/

(8) I've Got Some Good News and Some Bad News YOU'RE OLD. Tales of a Geriatrician: Bernstein, David MD
http://www.amazon.com/Ive-Got-Some-Good-News/dp/0990708705

Other Resources

Stern RA, D'Ambrosio LA, Mohyde M, Carruth A, Tracton-Bishop B, Hunter JC, Daneshvar DH, Coughlin JF. *At the crossroads: development and evaluation of a dementia caregiver group intervention to assist in driving cessation.* Gerontol Geriatr Educ. 2008;29(4) 363-382. doi:10.1080/02701960802497936. PMID: 19064472; PMCID: PMC2679525.

The Physician's Guide to Assessing and Counseling Older Drivers is available online at www.ama-assn.org or geriatricscareonline.org/ProductAbstract/physicians-guide-to-assessing-and-counseling-older-drivers/B013.

Suncoast Safety Council: CPR, OSHA, and Driver Training 1145 Court St. Clearwater, Florida 33756 (727)373-7233 Senior Drivers - Behind the Wheel Driving Lessons

CONTACT INFO

For further information or to reach David Bernstein, MD
Contact Media Dept.:
Melissa Bernstein, OTR/L, FAOTA
Publicist
Dynamic Learning/AGE GRACEFULLY®
813.855.2876 or via email at **Melissa@dynamicgrp.com**

Join in the conversation with Dr. Bernstein at:

> *Website:* www.davidbernsteinmd.com
> *Twitter:* https://twitter.com/DBernsteinMD
> *Facebook*: www.facebook.com/DavidBernsteinMD
> *LinkedIn:* http://www.linkedin.com/in/davidbernstein2200

GET MY FREE EBOOK-"NOTES ON LIVING LONGER"
www.davidbernsteinmd.com

About the Author

David Bernstein, MD is a highly respected physician who is board certified in both Internal Medicine and Geriatrics practicing in Clearwater, Florida. His 30 years of experience have provided him with opportunities to observe and empathize with thousands of adults as they age.

His compassion and ability to see the souls of his patients has compelled him to share his stories in his previously published book "*I've Got Some Good News and Some Bad News: YOU'RE OLD Tales of a Geriatrician...*"

Dr. Bernstein was motivated to share his thoughts about senior drivers after years of interacting with patients and their families.

He is a graduate of Washington University in St. Louis and Albany Medical College. He is an associate clinical professor in the department of medicine at the University of South Florida College Of Medicine.

Dr. Bernstein is an avid public speaker, addressing various medical topics with his colleagues and with the community at large with a focus on families facing the complex problems as they near the end of life.

Made in the USA
Middletown, DE
03 June 2022

66524051R00029